HARVEST LIVING

A Guided Devotional to Choosing Wellness

Menia "MJ" Johnson

Harvest Living: A Guided Devotional to Choosing Wellness © 2020 by Menia "MJ" Johnson. All Rights Reserved.

All rights reserved. No part of this book may be reproduced in any form or by any electronic or mechanical means including information storage and retrieval systems, without permission in writing from the author. The only exception is by a reviewer, who may quote short excerpts in a review.

Scripture quotations marked NIV are taken from The Holy Bible, New International Version®, NIV® Copyright © 1973, 1978, 1984, 2011 by Biblica, Inc.® Used by permission. All rights reserved worldwide.
Scripture quotations marked NKJV are taken from the New King James Version®. Copyright © 1982 by Thomas Nelson. Used by permission. All rights reserved.
Scripture quotations marked NLT are taken from the *Holy Bible*, New Living Translation, copyright © 1996, 2004, 2015 by Tyndale House Foundation. Used by permission of Tyndale House Publishers, Inc., Carol Stream, Illinois 60188. All rights reserved.

Cover designed by Avi Luxe Designs
Printed in the United States of America
First Printing: November 2020
The Scribe Tribe Publishing Group
Post Office Box 1264 Homewood, IL 60430

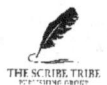
THE SCRIBE TRIBE
PUBLISHING GROUP

ISBN-13 978-1-7358251-4-4 (print)
ISBN-13 978-1-7358251-5-1 (electronic)

*To my past and your past for growing us
into greater days ahead.*

PREFACE

I am so honored to have the opportunity to share with you, as I have done with many in the recent past, a journey of healing the body emotionally, physically, and spiritually through a life of discipline in wellness. I began my own journey amid severe depression and wanting to just simply feel better about my life, my body, and have a mind that was regulated and well. Wellness can't be accomplished without inserting directives towards emotional and spiritual health. However, I do believe that with the three combined, the measure of sustainability for a lifetime of health is greater. This, my friend, is what I'd like to *call Harvest Living.* When in a time of harvest, we produce sustainable elements that drive our productivity and life forward for the greater. Now is your time. Every single day that you have breath in your body is an opportunity to live in wellness. So, before you begin this 21-day journey, I STRONGLY encourage you to have a journal (even if you choose to use a note app on your phone) nearby for extended writing. Consider, if you already haven't, taking advantage of a therapist/counselor, and invite your past, present, and future into this process.

Are you ready? Let's begin!

*YOU'VE CHOSEN DAY
ONE OF TWENTY-ONE!*

DAY ONE

Every day is day one.

My daytime job allows me to be surrounded by a team of men who listen to inspirational podcasts daily. The CEO of the company that I work for sent us that quote one day after we decided that a "re-set" was in order. We needed to focus our goals, initiatives, and plans towards a "day one" mentality.

Having a "day one" mentality means that you decide to have the same excitement, the same vigor, the same motivation of starting something new, every…single…day. This is how we should begin this journey of wellness. Sometimes, when we get "too far ahead of ourselves," as my mom used to say, we end up either not finishing or never really starting. The Bible tells us in Matthew 6:25 to not be concerned with what tomorrow will bring, because it already has a bunch of stuff to take care of. Of course, it doesn't say it exactly like that, but you get my drift!

Starting in of itself can be daunting. We must discover a pattern of not finishing before we begin yet another thing.

I remember being told that I was "too creative", and I needed to pick a lane because it appeared to that person that I was never really finishing. Now, the little attitude chick that I bury most of the time within the deepest part of my soul was super offended by that statement! Yes, yes! I was. I thought to myself, "You don't even know me...Why do you care so much... Stay in your lane sir!" But he was right! He had me take a moment and write out all the things I started, and either finished halfway or didn't give my all due to allowing myself to be pulled in many directions without instruction. Phew!

So, as I sat there doing the exercise, I realized that I have been blessed with many talents, but there is a season and a time for all of them. Doing them all well, at the same time, just wasn't a "thing" that I was able to master. After my list was completed, he had me to do a K.S.S. Graph. What is this, you ask? Well, let me tell you! **Keep. Start. Stop.**

Under each word, I needed to prioritize what I was going to focus on. If something landed in the stop column, it didn't mean that I was never to pick it up again. It just meant that I could place it there and move it to the start column when I knew I could complete it.

Today is your day one. Before we even get to the "lose weight" or eat well part of this journey, it is important that you discover other areas of your life where you've begun and never finished. Be honest and ask yourself a few questions. *Why did you begin? What happened in the middle? And why didn't you finish well or stay consistent.*

Today marks the beginning of a beautiful story and course correction that you are choosing. Take every thought captive. (2 Corinthians 10:5)

* * *

CAPTIVATE THE THOUGHTS OF YOUR PAST

1. What is your first memory of not finishing something?
2. How old were you?
3. What was the response from others (parents, friends, etc.) when you didn't finish?
4. How did you feel?

SURRENDER THEM NOW

God, I thank you for the lessons of my past. Help me to allow them to be only that and not a precursor for the rest of my life. I surrender my hurts and the triggers of my childhood or past relationships to You. Help me to honor myself by staying consistent moment by moment. Help me to choose myself and not my past.

Menia "MJ" Johnson

YOU'VE CHOSEN DAY TWO OF TWENTY-ONE!

DAY TWO

Do it well!

I have the belief that when I do something, I should do it well. In the past, well--who am I kidding?! Even present day, I put so much pressure on myself to do things well. Growing up, my dad used to encourage my siblings and I not to wait for tomorrow to do something great, and if we chose to do something, we should do it well. This ingredient of my life's recipe has taught me a sense of vigor that has proven itself well. However, at times, if I go all in without a plan to ensure that I execute, I fail. Failure always causes me to re-evaluate my original intentions.

When I started my personal journey of wellness, I would start and stop, gain, and then refrain from being honest with myself. It didn't dawn on me that it really began with my mind. It was not until I was able to admit to myself that there was a deeper-rooted issue of self-esteem and a disbelief that God cared about this part of my life that I was able to fully commit to my overall wellness and be disciplined.

Scripture encourages us to do all things to the Glory of God; ***"So whether you eat or drink, or whatever you do, do it all for the glory of God." 1 Corinthians 10:31 NLT***

I suppose we need to sit in what the "glory of God" really is when it comes to wellness.

Glory is the manifestation of God's presence. When we decide that we want to live in wellness, it is acknowledging that we want the manifestation of God's presence to embody our choices of caring for our bodies, minds, and souls.

Consider the *all* part of this scripture to also manifest itself within your food choices. When you feel the urge to have all the calories (i.e. pizza, fries, bad fatty foods, soda, nicotine, etc.), I want you to think about the scripture. Are you really glorifying God in your decision to bring unproductive foods into your system? Are you glorifying God in your decision to bring harm to your organs with abusing substances that degenerate your body? Are you glorifying God when you're choosing to repeat negative thought patterns because it's comfortable?

It only takes **one** moment, even one millisecond to choose wellness.

* * *

CAPTIVATE THE THOUGHTS OF YOUR PAST

1. What foods, choices, and/or mentalities do I currently have that harm my body?
2. What can I feasibly choose to give up today that will benefit my choice in wellness?

SURRENDER THEM NOW

God, thank You for another day of choosing wellness. Help me to be willing to acknowledge the food and things I've used to replace the moments You could have comforted me instead. I choose to live in full wellness with Your help and with the help of those around me.

* * *

***Manifest the Harvest – Try These!**_

HOME WORKOUT
25 Jumping Jacks
25 Squats
25 Mountain Climbers
25 High Knees (modifications are acceptable)
25 Ice Skaters
REPEAT 4x's
Minimal rest in between (30-45 seconds)

MJ's FAVORITE RECIPE #1
Cauliflower Bowl of Yummy

(It's my favorite easy meal prep and repeat dish.)
Ingredients: cauliflower rice; ground turkey; spinach; green onion; garlic; olive oil and roasted bell peppers

1. Drizzle a pan with olive oil.
2. Add your chopped green onion and garlic.
3. Add your frozen cauliflower rice.
4. Add raw spinach or frozen spinach.
5. Season with sea salt and pepper (or use seasoning of your choice with no carbs).
6. Cook for 15 minutes.
7. In a separate pan, brown and season 1 pound of ground turkey.
8. On the back eye of the stove (be sure it's clean lol), place two peppers to "roast." Cut in slices after you see the outside has turned black or looks burnt.
9. Mix your cooked ground turkey into the pan with your cauliflower mix.
10. Top with roasted peppers and enjoy.

Menia "MJ" Johnson

YOU'VE CHOSEN DAY THREE OF TWENTY-ONE!

DAY THREE

Resistance training is not just for working out.

Resistance training comes in to play for every area of our lives. Physically, we can use resistance bands to help strengthen our muscles while at home if we don't have actual weights. Emotionally, we can build boundaries in relationships and resist temptation when it comes around. And spiritually, we can choose to resist the enemy, lies, temptation, and doubt and he will flee from our decision-making processes.

For me, one of the greatest resistance lessons I had to learn was boundary setting in relationships with people and with food. To be honest, the food part was almost as hard as setting healthy relational boundaries.

If we're honest with ourselves, emotional eating typically happens because some human relationship has disturbed a portion of our brain! Be it work relationships, romantic relationships, bogus--I mean hard friendships *(insert nervous laughter here)*, or even familial relationships, someone or something has us overeating, grabbing the wine (Pinot Noir please!), and wallowing in emotional turmoil.

When choosing to live a life of wellness to include mental health, we literally must resist temptation at all costs. If you know that you have a weakness for unproductive food and relationships, consider starting with a choice to a) not have foods in your home that feed into lack of discipline and b) set internal boundaries for relationships that cause you anxiety or stress. Your choice of saying *no* is the ultimate resistance training.

It is a spiritual discipline that can feed into your physical and emotional life of wellness. **You can do this!**

The Bible says, ***"Submit yourselves then to God. Resist the devil, and he will flee from you." James 4:7 NIV***

Submit to God:
- Your food choices
- Your relationships
- Your job
- Boundaries that are productive

Resist:
- Negative thinking
- Bad relationships
- Emotional eating

* * *

CAPTIVATE THE THOUGHTS OF YOUR PAST

1. Who in my life has caused me the most stress? Is this a relationship that can be nurtured with boundaries and therapy?
2. What foods do I run to the most when I need to "feel better?"
3. Is there anything I need in addition to these steps to help me be more disciplined (ex. therapy, accountability, a plan)

SURRENDER THEM NOW

God, I thank You that You care for me. Thank You for helping me to resist unhealthy foods and relationships that cause me to be emotionally and physically unproductive. I thank You now for counselors, trainers, and accountability partners I currently have or that I plan to acquire soon. I acknowledge that You are with me in this and I am grateful for Your presence in this journey of full wellness. Amen.

YOU'VE CHOSEN DAY FOUR OF TWENTY-ONE!

DAY FOUR

You are a temple of purpose.

Yesterday, we learned about resistance training and ended the reflection by asking God to help us train our decisions and honor our bodies because it is where He lives.

Imagine your body being the very dwelling place of purpose, legacy, and honor. Seeing ourselves as a majestic temple, with an unshakeable foundation, creates in us a belief that we are well in every possible way.

There are days that I forget that I have a kingdom living within me. A kingdom, you ask? Yes, kingdom! A purposed life of legacy that holds the heart of God inside. I get caught up in what I must do, my kids, our family business, friendships, work, and life and I forget to take a moment to remember that I GET to live! I GET to make sure that the kingdom within is reflected on my outer body as well.

There is a scripture that I often meditate on that helps me to realign my body with the reality that God is within me and that I am completely capable of being sure my foundation, my core, my body is well. Philippians 1:6-7 indicates that if God started the work of forming me in my mother's womb and giving me purpose, He will be sure that that work is finished! What work? The work of me living in full wellness and full purpose with the kingdom He prepared for me in heaven and placed within me.

Every week that you decide to show up for yourself and choose the reality that your body is the temple of God here on earth, it is literally a decision that you've made to honor the price that was paid for your existence.

With every decision to eat well, drink your water and protect your mind, spirit, and relationships, you are honoring the temple of the Holy Spirit within you. How amazing is that?

"Don't you realize that your body is the temple of the Holy Spirit, who lives in you and was given to you by God? You do not belong to yourself, for God bought you with a high price. So you must honor God with your body." 1 Corinthians 6:19-20 NLT

* * *

CAPTIVATE THE THOUGHTS OF YOUR PAST

1. What negative thoughts have I had about my body?
2. When did that begin?
3. How can I honor my temple better starting today?

SURRENDER THEM NOW

Jesus, please help me to let go of the negative ideas I've had about the place in which You dwell, my body. Help me to realize that You created me in Your image and that because of You, I am. Thank You, now, that the deeply rooted issues from my past, even yesterday, are being plucked up each day of this journey until I am living a disciplined life of emotional, spiritual, and physical wellness. Amen.

* * *

Manifest the Harvest – Try These!
HOME WORKOUT

10 Push-ups (modifications are acceptable)
15 Shoulder Press
15 Bicep Curls
15 Triceps Kick Backs
10 Push-ups

REPEAT 4x's

Minimal rest in between (30-45 second)
Use laundry detergent if you don't have weights.

MJ's FAVORITE RECIPE #2
MJ's Low Carb Pancake Recipe

Ingredients: 2 large eggs, yolks and whites separated; 2 oz heavy whipping cream; 2 tsp erythritol granulated; pinch of sea salt; 2 oz almond flour; ¼ teaspoon baking powder (gluten free), 1 tsp unsalted butter

Yields 8 small pancakes

1. In a large mixing bowl, combine the egg yolks, whipping cream, low carb sweetener, and salt until the mixture is smooth.
2. In a small mixing bowl, combine almond flour with baking powder; whisk it into the creamy egg mixture until uniform in appearance.
3. Using an electric mixer, beat the egg whites in a separate bowl until soft peaks form. Fold the egg whites into the batter.
4. Melt butter in a large non-stick frying pan over medium heat, then wipe with a paper towel to evenly distribute the butter for cooking. Spoon in the batter to make your

pancakes; use about 2 tablespoons (30ml) per pancake.
5. Cook for 3 minutes, or until lightly browned, and then gently flip each pancake and cook for an additional 2 minutes on the other side. Take care not to agitate the pancake before it's ready to flip or disaster will ensue!

Menia "MJ" Johnson

YOU'VE CHOSEN DAY FIVE OF TWENTY-ONE!

DAY FIVE

Godly fitness is your guide to success.

"Physical training is good, but training for godliness is much better, promising benefits in this life and in the life to come." (1 Timothy 4:8 NLT) Many have been successful at being physically fit without growing spiritually. It has been done and will continue to be done. But you have chosen to accept the value in building your spiritual muscles as you concur the body and the mind.

Jesus wants your spirit to flourish during your time here on earth. Taking time to read the Bible, pray and meditate on the word of God ignites your faith in a way that mirrors growth (muscle gains) from lifting weights.

It is impossible for your relationship with Christ to grow if you aren't spending time with Him. Meditating on the words you read and asking Him to allow your mind to remember the things you've learned along the way are crucial to your spiritual development.

I remember being so confident that I was full of faith and knew Jesus for real until one day I realized I didn't really know Him for myself. I grew up as a pastor's kid, going to church almost seven days a week. For a while, that was enough. It wasn't taught initially that I was also to be reading the Bible outside of a Sunday service. Now, I am not saying that my foundation was not firm. I am saying that I only felt close to God when I was in fellowship with other believers on Sundays or at weekly gatherings. Then, I turned 15. I attended a youth group where the teenagers recited scripture, preached, and carried their own bibles! Like, their own bibles that they brought from home and not the pew bibles! These kids were praying scripture and living in Christ, not by Christ. *I. Was. Blown. Away!*

That is when I started reading the Bible and praying in my bedroom. I felt closer to God, in a room by myself for the first time. This is when I knew what relationship with Him felt like.

As you grow spiritually fit, remember that you don't have to be surrounded by others to "feel" the presence of God. You do have to spend time learning His promises, His heart, and His will. This can only be done by intentionally choosing time(s) during your day that is only for you and Him. For some, this sounds like a daunting task! But there are so many online tools that can get you started. Check out online Bible plans, online bibles, YouTube channels, etc.

Set an alarm. Rise. Pray. Sit in His presence. Live in Him.

* * *

CAPTIVATE THE THOUGHTS OF YOUR PAST

1. What lies have I told myself about why I can't be spiritually fit?
2. Where did these ideas begin?
3. What do I need to unlearn to be disciplined in my spiritual fitness?
4. How has a lack of faith affected my mental health?

SURRENDER THEM NOW

Dear Jesus, thank You for Your grace and mercy towards me. According to 2 Corinthians 12:9, Your power is made perfect in my weaknesses. I appreciate Your grace and power in my life as You are renewing my mind, spirit, and soul towards wellness. It is Your promise to be with me, and not forsake me, even in this. Forgive me for neglecting the reality of Your power within me. Amen.

YOU'VE CHOSEN DAY
SIX OF TWENTY-ONE!

DAY SIX

Control yourself!

Control and discipline. These words are like twin brothers...two peas in a pod...besties even! Many believe that it takes 21 days to create a habit, but it is also said that it takes three cycles of 21 days to truly be transformed in the mind. Let's do some math shall we? That is 63 days! A little over two months. 1,512 hours of choosing a new way of thinking. Good goodness, that seems like a really long time doesn't it? Yes! Yes, it does.

But guess what? It really isn't in comparison to how long Noah was on an ark with all those animals and some people too! Before he even began sailing the world, he had to BUILD the ark. He had to control his human impulses to give up, delay the process, or even grow weary in what he knew God called him to do. Imagine him getting to week two of the building process and deciding that it was just too much to do? Or, that it wasn't worth all the hard work because he didn't trust that he could finish the assignment he was ordained to do? I believe that what we know as the world would look completely different, or maybe not even exist. Is this a stretch of the imagination? Maybe! But it gives us a bit of perspective in this amazing journey to wellness. Things will not happen overnight, neither will our ability to live a disciplined life. We must first begin with controlling our minds. The things we tell ourselves become truths when they are really lies that will eat away at our designed purpose to live well.

    I remember I used to tell myself that smoking wasn't such a bad habit. I started smoking at a very young age and it was a habit that I let control my emotions. It was something I CHOSE to do when stress would come about. I told myself that I "needed" to smoke. It was "time to myself" in an alley somewhere, with a spray bottle of body splash to hide the smell. We entrap ourselves in the lack of discipline when we choose to lie that we "need" something that isn't fruitful to our bodies, minds, and spirits. It may not be smoking for you though. It may be sweet treats, sex outside of marriage, pornography, drinking, elongated sleeping time, or even laziness masked as resting.

1 Corinthians 9:27 encourages us to discipline our body and keep it under control. You can control your actions to create a lifestyle of discipline! It is simply how God intended you to live.

* * *

CAPTIVATE THE THOUGHTS OF YOUR PAST

1. What physical things do I need to surrender that are weighing me down emotionally?
2. When did my lack of controlling my desires begin? Was it when I was a child, teen, or adult?
3. How can I begin to captivate my thoughts of destruction emotionally and physically starting today?

SURRENDER THEM NOW

Heavenly Father, I know that I cannot begin to gain control over my thought life or wellness until I give You control. Help me to manifest productivity into my life by choosing to control my desires. Thank You now for delivering me from the hand of the enemies I've chosen in the past. Help me to rely only on You to gain control of my mind, my spirit, and my body. I welcome change today. I welcome surrender. Amen.

* * *

Manifest the Harvest – Try These!

HOME CARDIO WORKOUT
25 Jump Squats (modifications are acceptable)
20 Skaters
20 Mountain Climbers
25 Jumping Jacks (modifications are acceptable)
60 Seconds of Running in Place
REPEAT 4x's
Minimal rest in between (30-45 second)

MJ's Favorite Recipe #3
Fajita Bowl

Ingredients: 4 cups of brown rice (1 cup per meal); 4 mixed colored bell peppers; 1 medium yellow onion; 1-16 oz can of black beans; 1 pound of ground turkey; 2 limes; Mrs. Dash Chipotle seasoning; Mrs. Dash Garlic & Herb seasoning; 1 pack of low sodium taco seasoning; black pepper

1. Heat oven to 375 degrees.
2. Oil a sheet pan.

3. Cut peppers and onions into slices, season with a packet of low sodium taco seasoning and black pepper, drizzle with olive oil and roast in the oven for 30 minutes.
4. Heat canned black beans and season with 2 teaspoons of Mrs. Dash Chipotle seasoning.
5. Cook brown rice and add a pinch of salt (literally) and squeeze lime in when it is done. Stir well.
6. Brown ground turkey season with Mrs. Dash Garlic & Herb seasoning and a bit of black pepper.
7. Prep your bowls/containers: 1 cup of brown rice, 1 cup of veggies, ½ cup of black beans and 1 cup of ground turkey.

Menia "MJ" Johnson

YOU'VE CHOSEN DAY SEVEN OF TWENTY-ONE!

DAY SEVEN

Work out your worship.

This may sound completely bananas, but did you know, or have you ever considered that working out is worship? You're probably like, "what in the world is MJ talking about?" Well, I am going to tell you now, it is!

Consider the scripture ***Romans 12:1: And so, dear brothers and sisters, I plead with you to give your bodies to God because of all he has done for you. Let them be a living and holy sacrifice—the kind he will find acceptable. This is truly the way to worship him.***

It says it in there! If you are *intentional* about what you eat, drink, and how you choose to move your body daily, it is considered worship unto the Lord. Our lives already have the opportunity to be a life of worship.

But let's define, or shall I say redefine, what worship really is. I think we get so caught up in the "church" definition of worship thinking that it is only a song that we sing that may possibly have a slower melody than that of a "praise" song which is often considered to be more upbeat. Worship is defined as the feeling or expression of reverence and adoration for a deity. *Expression.* Let's sit in this word for a bit, shall we?

Expression is the *process* of making known one's thoughts or feelings.

Your choice in wellness is this process, friend. The process of discipline. The process of committing to a workout regimen. The process of healing your mind from unproductive thinking. The process of healing your heart from past traumas.

The intentional process.

I remember being in a place that I wished for my life to be a life of worship and thought I had to walk around singing all the time. That isn't such a horrible thing since I really do love to sing. However, I knew that it was meant to be something else. After weeks, months, even years of trying to figure this worship life out, I realized that my fitness journey was this! Now that was an epic moment for me, friend!

It is one of the reasons you've chosen to participate in finishing this devotional. I wanted to be sure that you too knew that this lifestyle is worship unto the Lord.

You sacrifice time. You sacrifice a good, yummy, high-caloric, sodium-filled meal. You choose to delight yourself in productive behaviors when you intentionally choose to live this lifestyle as worship.

I am already so proud of you. But God is even honored by your sacrifices. That is amazing!

So, before we rid ourselves of some things, I want to encourage you to remember what you've read today. Challenge yourself to see every workout, every healthy meal eaten, and therapy as an act of worship.

Maybe even play some uplifting Jesus music while you're getting it in! (I personally love the artist Lecrae or hip-hop Jesus tunes to get me going.)

* * *

CAPTIVATE THE THOUGHTS OF YOUR PAST

1. In what ways have I denied my soul and spirit an atmosphere of worship?
2. What or who do I need to sacrifice today that is causing me to pull away from this journey of wellness?
3. What productive choice can I make today that can be an expression of my worship unto God?

SURRENDER THESE NOW

God, I thank You for this new lifestyle of worship. I dedicate my food choices, my therapy appointments, and my physical fitness to you as an acceptable and pleasing sacrifice. Thank You for every drip of sweat!

Thank You for every well digested food choice I make today. Thank You for my accountability circle who are constantly encouraging me to keep going. But most of all, thank You for being with me every step of the way. I surrender my past to You. I surrender my brokenness to You, and I receive Your grace and mercy. For it is by Your grace, that I am saved. Amen.

Menia "MJ" Johnson

YOU'VE CHOSEN DAY EIGHT OF TWENTY-ONE!

DAY EIGHT

You need hydrated strength for the journey.

Have you ever been so incredibly thirsty and gulped down a bottle of water in epic time? I know I have.

I remember running, well let's be honest, jogging my first 5k. It was warm and I was so stinking thirsty and could not wait for the water station. I didn't know that I could drink water so fast and be so appreciative for the ability to swallow! In real life! It was like I had never had water before a day in my life.

I hope that over this last week you've learned the importance of hydration. Not just physically, but spiritually. This process of learning a new lifestyle comes with challenging days where you'll feel weary. You may even experience moments that you want to give up because you aren't seeing the results you hoped for.

Isaiah 40:31* says, *"But they who wait upon the Lord, shall renew their strength; they shall mount up on eagles; they shall run, and not be weary; they shall walk and not faint." (KJV) Let me be clear: weariness can come from a lack of hydration, friend.

Physically, if we are not consuming at least a gallon of water a day, especially if we've been intentional about working out, our muscles become fatigued. Our body cannot function well if we are giving it the simple gift of water!

Weariness in spirit comes if we aren't giving our souls the water of life--the word of God.

Now, I understand if you may not be a "Bible thumper," which is not necessarily the call of God. It is, however, a necessary component of growing spiritual muscles. How can we know Him if we do not read about Him, His promises, stories of faith, and correction? How can we really grow in our spiritual walk if we aren't doing any kind of spiritual lifting outside of begging--*I mean praying*--every now and again? We can't.

Hydrate your spirit and gain the strength, wisdom, and discipline you need to attack your goals and live in full wellness.

If you're new to the whole Bible deal, I encourage you to order a translation that is easy for you to understand. Try either the Message Bible, Christian English Bible, or even the New Living Translation. If you're not a "paper book" kind of person, that is ok! Hello technology! Check out the Bible App. There are literally a kajillion (*not a real word*) versions in that app and even some Bible plans that can kick you off into a great beginning.

If you are a "seasoned saint" and have been reading the Bible for ages, there's something new for you too! Challenging yourself to dive into a book of the Bible that you haven't read in a while is the place to start. For me, I realized that the books of Jonah, Micah, Nahum, and even Zephaniah were not my go-to reads! However, there are some major life lessons and great teachings of faith and discipline there. Don't take for granted your years of faith. There is ALWAYS a new level God intends for us for we are to grow in faith, from faith to faith. (Romans 1:17)

* * *

CAPTIVATE THE THOUGHTS OF YOUR PAST

1. How have I been depriving myself from spiritual hydration?
2. Do I have any hang ups on drinking water? Why? What can I do to increase my intake?
3. Outside of my body being weary from my new workout regimen, what/who else is weighing me down?
4. What do I need to do to stay mentally and spiritually hydrated so that I do not grow increasingly weary?

SURRENDER THESE NOW

Jesus, please forgive me for allowing my spirit and body to become complacent. Help me to realize the importance of the simple gift of water. The water from the earth and the water from your endless river of life. Thank You that I am growing in faith and as I grow, I become stronger. Help me to lay aside any relational weight (burden), mindsets, or laziness that is depriving me from strength all together. I commit my life to You today, Lord. Amen.

* * *

Manifest the Harvest – Try These!

HOME WORKOUT
20 Bicep Curls
(use laundry detergent if you don't have weights)
20 Upright Rows
25 Jumping Jacks
10 Push-ups
20 Sit-ups
REPEAT 4x's
Minimal rest in between (30-45 seconds)

MJ's Favorite Recipe #4
Rooted Veggies

Ingredients: 1 bag of carrots; 3 sweet potatoes; 2 parsnips; 2 beet bulbs; 1 bunch of fresh parsley; 3 garlic bulbs; 1 small red onion; 3-4 oz chicken breasts; olive oil, balsamic dressing; salt and pepper

1. Heat oven to 425.
2. Dice all veggies into cubes.

3. Oil a large sheet pan.
4. Spread your cubed veggies on the pan and drizzle balsamic dressing and olive oil over the top and place parsley and garlic bulbs between the veggies. Roast for 30-40 minutes.
5. Sauté your chicken and season with lite salt & pepper. Feel free to use Mrs. Dash Garlic seasoning.
6. Prep your containers: 2 cups of veggies and your protein.

Menia "MJ" Johnson

YOU'VE CHOSEN DAY NINE OF TWENTY-ONE!

DAY NINE

You can win the anxiety battle.

You may have never experienced any anxiety before in your life. Perhaps, you are always calm, never worried, full of optimism and live a carefree life.

On the other hand, although I grew up in a calm household without much confrontation, I grew into an adult with a mind full of wonder and worry. The "what if" mentality definitely became stronger than the "I can handle anything" mentality.

When initially beginning my journey and then starting over time and time again, I was full of "*what if* this doesn't work" and "*I can't handle* this level of commitment" type of thinking. I am certain that I told myself millions of times that I am too much of a free-spirited chick to willingly stick to a lifestyle of wellness. *What if* I get injured? *What if* I can't get to the gym because of the kids' schedules? *I can't handle* the soreness. *I can't handle* eating something I'm not used to digesting.

See, anxiety doesn't always necessarily mean that we have an issue that comes with the idea of needing physiological help. Anxiety can be an unintentional learned behavior we allow in our lives as normal thinking. What I've divulged about my past thought patterns really came from childhood rooted issues of not knowing how to deal with confrontation. I did not really understand that my inability to confront myself and my mind about my unwillingness to commit to my wellness was a process of unlearning thought patterns and behaviors.

How could I possibly confront the negative thoughts if I was uncomfortable with all confrontation? Not possible!

Now that you've had a moment to think differently about the word *anxiety*, maybe you too need to unlearn some thought patterns you've created over time.

Philippians 4:6* encourages us to *"Be anxious for nothing, but in everything by prayer and supplication, with thanksgiving, let your requests be made known to God..." (NKJV)

So, as you CHOOSE everyday of this devotional and prayerfully the days following these, remember to bring up anything to God. Ask Him to help you change the way you talk to yourself! Ask Him to assist you in the training of truthful speech and actionable responses that will be fruitful to your new disciplined life. He really does care about it all.

* * *

CAPTIVATE THE THOUGHTS OF YOUR PAST

1. What stories (lies) have I told myself about eating well or exercise?
2. What have I thought about yourself if I wanted to go to therapy?
3. What are some of the things I remember from my childhood that may play a part in how I think?
4. Who in my life, either present or past, has ever told me 'no' or that I couldn't achieve a goal? *(Even if you were that person, write it down.)*

SURRENDER THEM NOW

Heavenly Father, You are my strength, my protector, and the regulator of my mind. I thank You now that You are creating within me, inwardly and on the outside, a strong disciplined person. Thank You for the knowledge of Your word and the words of this devotional that are helping me to dig deep, surrender, and live a life of full wellness. I pray that I will retain words from this Harvest devotional that filtrate all my days. Amen.

YOU'VE CHOSEN DAY TEN OF TWENTY-ONE!

DAY TEN

You are wonderfully made.

If you have ever been to church or had a "churchie" friend, I am sure that you've heard the scripture this day is entitled after. If you haven't let me share it with you.

"I will praise You, for I am fearfully and wonderfully made; Marvelous are Your works, And that my soul knows very well." Psalm 139:14 NKJV

Now, if you're like me and have been on a journey of fitness and wellness for a while, you may often look in the mirror and struggle to believe that you are wonderfully made. The mirror reflects what we sometimes do not want to see! Let's be honest, shall we? Yes? Yes.

I can vividly remember making myself stand in the mirror naked at the beginning of my wellness journey, embracing what I saw staring back at me. That was one of the hardest "self-care" moments of my life. Choosing to recite this scripture to a woman, *me*, that I didn't feel comfortable with. I recited this scripture until I let it sink into my spirit, my mind, and my soul. No, I wasn't looking at abs or defined arms. I was looking at a few rolls, flabby arms, and a sad woman who had faced several relational traumas. I wasn't down on myself fully because I was not fit. I was down on myself because, for some years, I didn't think that I was enough. Enough for me, for a man, for solid friendships, for happiness even.

All this trauma translated into overeating, lots of cocktails, a few, well, many packs of Newport cigarettes, and a body that took in all the things to give me momentary comfort. It wasn't until I chose to realize that I was created in the image of God that I was able to release the traumas and embrace this truth of being wonderfully made. That's when discipline showed up to stay.

Will it take some time? *Yes.* Is it worth it? *Yes.*

You, my friend, are also wonderfully made. Your soul longs to hold on to this truth for the rest of your days here on earth.

Today is another day to do the hard work.

Are you hoping that I don't encourage you to stand naked in front of the mirror? Well, I totally am!

This practice has become a daily choice for me. It is liberating, it is hard, it is really the naked truth. No more hiding from your emotions or heartache, trauma, or disappointments. God already sees you. Now is the time for you to see yourself fully. See and acknowledge the parts of you that you absolutely love, even if it's the corner of your elbows! This process will also allow you to say aloud the inner parts of you that you are surrendering during this process of living a full circle wellness lifestyle.

How to do this practice:
- Write down Psalm 139:14 on a notecard and place it in your bathroom or a mirror in your bedroom.
- Stand in that mirror naked.
- Recite the scripture.
- State 2-3 things that you love about what you see.
- State 2-3 things that you want God's healing power to rectify outwardly or inwardly. (This can be anything.)
- Say to yourself "I am made in the image of God. He is my strength. He is my source. He is with me today as I choose to eat well, live well, and live in His grace." (Write this on another notecard.)

* * *

CAPTIVATE THE THOUGHTS OF YOUR PAST

1. What have I told myself about my body?
2. Are these thoughts positive or negative?
3. Have I done the mirror exercise before? If yes, how did that make me feel? If not, what is my greatest fear in doing this practice?
4. Has anyone ever body shamed me? If yes, how did that make me feel?

SURRENDER THESE NOW

God, I thank You that I am learning to accept the body You've given me. Thank You for helping me live in full wellness and not in shame. I pray that as I choose to eat well, exercise, and maybe even seek counsel, that You are with me every step of the way. I surrender those who have made me feel bad about myself. I choose today to release them from the prison of my heart, so that I can live in freedom and the fact that You have created me wonderfully and in Your image. My body will respond to wellness. My soul will respond to freedom and grace. My mind will be free of negative thinking. All because of Your grace and favor upon my life. Amen.

YOU'VE CHOSEN DAY ELEVEN OF TWENTY-ONE!

DAY ELEVEN

Just do it.

The great news is that as you work towards your goals physically, emotionally, and spiritually and do this work as unto God, it will naturally spill over into your relationships.

You're not doing any of this work for anyone else but as honor unto God. But as you honor Him, those around you will be blessed by seeing your dedication and testimony. You have not stayed committed for the last eleven days just for the compliments (*but they sure do feel good)!* The goal of this devotional is for you to be transformed fully for today, tomorrow and the days to come.

When we decide that we are worth it, those around us benefit from our choice of disciplined living.

Doing the hard work of getting to the root of our emotional and spiritual issues will reflect in our wellness journey. The Bible encourages us in Colossians 3:23 to work heartily for the Lord and not for man. Our choices to eat foods that are productive for our bodies, inwardly and outwardly, is like a gift to God.

Why do I say this? I believe with all my heart that God has provided us an opportunity to live in health with the simple choices of eating foods that bring healing to our bodies. So many diseases can be rectified with a combination of faith AND food. From joint pain to cancer, diabetes, fibroids and many more.

The saying "Just do it" can be intimidating at first. Thoughts of failure, letting people down, it being too hard, and the gamut of "what ifs" flood the mind.

This is where that faith initiative comes in. This is where getting to the root of your own disbelief system comes in. This is where you get to decide if your spirit is stronger than the negative parts of your mind that have driven the vehicle of unproductive living all these years.

When we've really decided that our full wellness is the key to breaking generational curses, thinking, and patterns, the doing becomes our champion of success.

You, my friend, can and will do this!

Choose every single day that you will receive the goodness of the Lord in the land of the living. (Psalm 27:13)

What is this goodness? Health. A sound mind. Reconciliation between you, the Lord, and others. Freedom.

* * *

CAPTIVATE THE THOUGHTS OF YOUR PAST

1. How many times have I started something and not finished?
2. Did I see my parents/adult influences execute goals successfully? If no, how did that impact my patterns of unproductivity?
3. Do I feel negative pressure to finish projects or execute my goals? Why?

SURRENDER THEM NOW

Dear God, I release myself from the negative pressures of life right now. I receive Your grace in this moment. I receive Your power through the Holy Spirit to activate the anointing of executing my wellness goals effectively and efficiently. I choose today to do the hard work. I choose today to uproot every generational pattern of slothfulness, disease, rather physical or mental, lack of execution and spiritual emptiness. I receive the fullness of joy from You and I expect to see results from the productive choices I will make daily. Thank You for leading me and guiding me into full wellness. Amen.

* * *

Manifest the Harvest – Try These!

HOME CARDIO WORKOUT
25 Jumping Jacks
1-minute Running in Place (quickly)
25 Burpees
25 Skaters
1-minute High Knees
REPEAT 4x's
Minimal rest in between (30-45 second)

MJ's Favorite Recipe #5
Spicy Sweet Potato Bowl

Ingredients: 6 small, sweet potatoes; 5 broccoli crowns; 1 pound of lean ground turkey (or protein of choice); Mrs. Dash Chipotle seasoning; minced garlic in olive oil; crushed red pepper flakes; dash of salt/pepper

1. Heat your oven to 375 degrees.

2. Peel your sweet potatoes and cut into cubes.
3. Oil a sheet pan and spread your sweet potatoes out on the pan. Season with Mrs. Dash Chipotle seasoning and just a pinch of salt and pepper.
4. Roast for 30 minutes.
5. While that is cooking, heat a large skillet and placed the minced garlic, ground turkey, red pepper flakes, salt, and pepper into the pan. Cook until the ground turkey is browned.
6. In a separate pot, simply steam your broccoli.
7. Now prep your bowls: 6 oz of ground turkey,1 cup of sweet potatoes, 1 cup of broccoli. Store until you're ready to eat.

Menia "MJ" Johnson

YOU'VE CHOSEN DAY TWELVE OF TWENTY-ONE!

DAY TWELVE

You're so swole!

I used to--well, who am I kidding? I *still* scroll Instagram and look at photos of fitness athletes trying to get an idea of how I'd like my body to look one day.

Sometimes it pumps me all the way up, and other days, I look at myself in the mirror and realize how much more work I really have to do. I am grateful for my "mirror moments" where I remind myself that I am fearfully and wonderfully made.

Comparison is the enemy to successful living, my friend. It is totally ok to glean from those who have successfully manifested their goals or initiatives. However, be sure that the gleaning is for learning and motivation only. When we compare ourselves to other people, we lose perfect moments to realize how powerful we are just being ourselves. The power we as an individual possess can never be measured against another human who has a different journey than we do.

Our strength comes from God. ***Proverbs 24:5*** encourages us to remember that ***"A wise man/woman is strong. Yes, a man/woman of knowledge increases strength." (NKJV)***

As we journey together and learn the tools of strength we need for full circle wellness, the wisdom we receive is a gift. This gift of knowledge and surrender is what will make us stronger.

So, when you think of being super "swole," even if that is not your goal, think of being full of strength in mind, body, and spirit. I also want to remind you to intentionally think of yourself that way when you feel weak and aren't considering your inner strength. When fear comes, or the "I don't feel like it" raises up, God is with you. He can and desires to be your strength.

You may wonder how you can allow God to be your strength? How is this a practical thing when you can't see Him? When He isn't the "trainer" helping you with your workout routine or the "chef" in your kitchen helping you to make good food decisions. Or even the "counselor" you may see on occasion? How does this really, practically work in today's world?

Well, my friends, simply put--trust. Trust the relationship you're building with the Most High God. When you dedicate time reading your Bible, praying, and pausing/yielding before making decisions of strength, you become stronger in faith. You become strong enough to trust the God who has created you. This practice of trusting God takes as much time as it does build muscle. Be willing to be undone in the presence of God during this process of full circle wellness. He is with you.

* * *

CAPTIVATE THE THOUGHTS OF YOUR PAST

1. What habits have I been accustomed to that showed my weaknesses? (i.e. emotional eating, negative thought processes, etc.)
2. Have I ever compared myself to others in a negative way? Why have I allowed myself to stay in this mindset?
3. Do I believe that I'm capable of changing negative habits?

SURRENDER THEM NOW

Heavenly Father, I believe that Your word says that I can cast all my anxiety upon You. You said that You'd carry my burdens when I am weak. I acknowledge my many moments of weakness and receive Your strength today. Help me to believe that You are my strength, my source, my trainer, my chef, and my counselor. I admit that there have been times that I may not have trusted You fully. Today, I receive You in a new way. I come to You broken, ready to be healed, and ready to be full of trust in Your promise to never leave me or forsake me. Today, my strength and trust are in You and I thank You for the changes that I have made and will continue to make. Amen.

Menia "MJ" Johnson

YOU'VE CHOSEN DAY THIRTEEN OF TWENTY-ONE!

DAY THIRTEEN

Get the revelation of rest.

I am the first to admit that resting wasn't at the top of my list. Napping is and has always been a part of my life, but even in the physical "rest" that I enjoy, I have had to learn to rest in mind and spirit as well. This, my friend, is the hardest part of living.

Learning to literally lay aside the day's worries, stresses, frustrations, disappointments and even joys before laying ourselves to bed at night is another muscle we must rain.

I can remember, even recently, being restless in my sleep. I am sure that I am not the only one that has experienced this. I couldn't stop thinking about all the work I had to do or what went wrong the day before. *What could I have done differently? Were my words expressed correctly during moments of confrontation? Why don't I do well with confrontation? How am I going to be able to parent children during a pandemic (this is being written during the summer of COVID-19)? Am I really doing all I can to define my body the way it needs to developed before the fall?*

See? My mind, and I am sure yours at times, goes a million miles a minute, even when we are laying down. So, how do we really rest in the Lord when we are these human beings with a ton of stuff going on?

How will our muscles recover when we desire to keep going during our workouts daily trying to hit a new goal or milestone?

Why is this important thing called rest such an integral part of living?

Rest, my friend, brings healing to our bodies, our souls, and our minds. Matthew 11:28-30 tells us that when we are weary, God will give us rest. He can only really give us what we desire, what we welcome.

It isn't a wonder that trainers and fitness experts encourage taking one or two rest days to allow our muscles to recover from our workout routines. This idea is not a man-made idea. It is a God idea! He loves us just that much to include it in the instructions written in the Bible. How amazing is God, right? He wants us to rest, not just sleep our lives away, but allow our spirits and minds to rest while He works on eternal life.

* * *

CAPTIVATE THE THOUGHTS OF YOUR PAST

1. Have I ever gone to bed and awakened tired? If so, what were the primary reasons for this?
2. What evening habits can I form to ensure that my mind can be at rest? (examples: journaling, turning off my phone, no TV, etc.)

3. What day(s) of the week can I commit to resting physically? What measures will I take to ensure this happens?

SURRENDER THEM NOW

Dear God, forgive me for the many times I've allowed my body and mind to be consumed by the things of this world to the point of exhaustion. Help me to remember that You want me to rest. Thank You now for the foods, daily productive habits, and measures I'll be taking that will give me more time to rest. I thank You also for the times where the extended time awake is full of purpose. Help me to never take for granted the time You've given me to succeed, or the time You've given me to rest. I receive Your joy, peace and grace going forward. Amen.

* * *

Manifest the Harvest – Try These!

HOME CARDIO WORKOUT
25 Plank Jacks (oh yeah!)
25 Standing Knee to Opposite Elbow
25 High Knees
25 Mountain Climbers
25 Squat & Shoulder Press (use weights or bands)
REPEAT 4x's
Minimal rest in between (30-45 second)

MJ's Favorite Recipe #6
Lemon Lime Salmon & Asparagus

Ingredients: 1 large salmon filet; 2 bunches of asparagus; 2 large lemons; Tajin seasoning (Aldi); minced garlic; black pepper; olive oil; pink salt; dried basil

1. Turn your oven broiler on high.
2. Prep your salmon: Use 2 tablespoons of minced garlic and spread over your salmon. Press it into the salmon with your fingertips.

Sprinkle Tajin, dry basil, and pepper over the salmon.

3. Broil for 10-15 minutes (Do not overcook it and dry it out.) Squeeze juice from one lemon over the salmon when it's done.
4. In a skillet on top of the stove, crisp your asparagus (Be sure to cut off the end of the stalk and then cut asparagus in half.) Heat skillet with olive oil and add your asparagus, pink salt, pepper, and juice from your second lemon. Cook for no more than 5-7 minutes. Your asparagus should be vibrant green.
5. Prep your bowls: 1 to 2 cups of asparagus on the bottom and top with 4 oz of salmon

YOU'VE CHOSEN DAY FOURTEEN OF TWENTY-ONE!

DAY FOURTEEN

Will He? Or won't He?

So, I was raised in a very charismatic church setting. Oftentimes, songs became scripture more than the scripture itself. I remember hearing time and time again that "God wouldn't give me more than I could bear," and in those times, it felt like He gave me a lot more than I could handle!

How was I to trust what I was learning, hearing, and singing but didn't "feel" like it was true? How was I supposed to believe that God really cared enough about the details of my life that He wouldn't let me get to the point of feeling super sad. He is God, right? He can see me freaking out. He can see the things that are going on in my life. He can see me binge eating in the lot of Wendy's before picking up my children from daycare. Yes?

Something happened in my journey to figure out if what I grew up believing was true. I decided to Google it! And low and behold, the scriptures really DON'T say that! I may or may not have needed a little therapy from the reality that maybe this wasn't the only thing I grew up believing that wasn't true. But I digress.

"No temptation <u>has overtaken you</u> except what is common to mankind. And God is faithful; he will not <u>let you be tempted beyond what you can bear</u>. But when you are tempted, he will also provide a way out <u>so that you can endure it</u>." 1 Corinthians 10:31 NIV

When I began this wellness journey, I knew that it was going to have to be more than just a diet. I had to start with my mind, my heart, my habits, my routines, and my belief systems.

The scripture indicates that what we go through isn't uncommon for many. The temptations we face are within our abilities to control ONLY when we decide that we have CHOICES. We can choose to live a productive life, or a life that is undisciplined.

A way out can simply be starting with therapy. Then, cutting out one unproductive habit a month versus trying to eliminate a lifetime of bad habits in 21 days (including this devotional). We each must decide what is within our own ability and if we need accountability until we can see for ourselves what we are capable of.

Emotional eating, casual sex, alcoholism, lying, stealing, and bad stewardship of finances are all a choice we use as a coping mechanism for something that is missing in our lives.

Often, it is a combination of a lack of external and internal love from others and ourselves that leads us into unproductive living.

Today, you get to decide if you're willing to see just what you're capable of. You get to decide what is within your own newly transformed "ability."

If there is lack, know that there are resources and people who are waiting to see you succeed! Support groups, churches, therapists, and maybe even friends who are on the same journey.

You can endure this process. With Christ, this is possible. How? Because it is His desire that your soul (heart) not perish. God really does want to see you live a productive lifestyle that includes full circle wellness. You just have to decide if you're willing to lay aside your old thought patterns to begin. Are you?

* * *

CAPTIVATE THE THOUGHTS OF YOUR PAST

1. What are some things I grew up believing to be true that I later found out weren't? Have these things aided in how I treat my body or spirit?
2. What unproductive habit do I have in my life today that I can honestly say I am tired of?
3. Who in my circle of friends or family do I trust to tell this to? If there is no one, will I consider seeking a therapist? If no, why?

SURRENDER THEM NOW

God, I thank You for teaching me the simplicity of the inspired word of Your heart. Help me to be willing to have my mind transformed through knowledge from the Bible, truth from those who know You well, and through my own ability to accept change. I repent now for choosing habits that have been unproductive in my life. I receive peace in my mind, my blood system, my heart, and anything else that has kept my life unaligned to Your will. I look forward to choosing, enduring, and living a discipline life. Amen.

YOU'VE CHOSEN DAY FIFTEEN OF TWENTY-ONE!

DAY FIFTEEN

Disable the disability.

Now, when we see the word *disability*, we may quickly think of someone who has a visible physical disability. Although this could be true, let's dig deeper into the reality that we may also have a disability.

Before you give me the side eye or your eyebrow raises in thought like, "What are you trying to say, MJ," I want you to be open while choosing today's devotional and exercise.

Let's say you do have a physical ailment; how many times have you said to yourself, "I can't do that because of XYZ reasons?" or "There is no way that I will be able to accomplish. . .?" Although there may be some things that are physically impossible, there are always modifications to physical exercises to keep your body strong. However, if your mind isn't as strong or your faith hasn't been fortified, you won't ever be able to get over the thoughts of being "unable."

When we've told ourselves for so long that we are incapable of achieving a goal or doing something super hard, it is no wonder that we get stuck or bogged down. Our thought patterns then become our disability.

When we continuously choose unproductive thinking, our bodies respond to what we think.

Proverbs 23:7 states, ***"For as he thinks in his heart, so is he." (NKJV)*** I am sure that we would never use the word "disabled" to characterize ourselves. However, our language, our decisions to deliberately not try, or our negative responses to stress become what disables us friends.

I have seen so many days of not being able to physically move. When I had my first stroke years ago, physical therapy was such a challenge. I remember laying on the mat trying to tell my mind to tell my legs to move and nothing would happen. There was a moment, though, that my heart had to decide that the foundation of my faith was stronger than my mind. At the end of that week, I remember my heart being full of what I knew to be true. I made Deuteronomy 31:8 personal! "It is the Lord who goes before me. He will be with me. He will never forsake me, so I will not be dismayed."

In that moment, my heart told my mind to tell my legs to move. You see, there are some who say, "mind over matter," but what happens when your mind has been trained to believe the opposite because of continual negative thinking?

God is the one who created our minds to function. *We can never allow an illusion of will power to take away the wealth of what faith can and will always be able to accomplish.*

Let us choose today to disable our physical and mental disabilities. Today, we will choose to allow God to renew our minds through the knowledge the

Bible brings to us and by our faith as we trust Him in the days ahead.

* * *

CAPTIVATE THE THOUGHTS OF YOUR PAST

1. What negative thought patterns have disabled me in the past?
2. Where did these thought patterns begin?
3. How can I actively choose to have productive thinking in the days ahead (journaling, praying, counseling, etc.)?
4. Who was the first person that told me that I couldn't do something? How did that impact you as a child and now as an adult?

SURRENDER THEM NOW

God, forgive me for the days and moments that I chose my own will over the truth of who You are. Help me to be willing to have my mind transformed as I grow in knowledge of the Gospel, tangible truths, and the disablement of my past. Today, I choose to believe that You will never forsake me. Today I choose to believe that You care about my physical, spiritual, and emotional well-being. Help me to forgive those who have punctured my thought patterns with negative speech. Replace my current thought patterns with truths so that I can live in wellness. Thank You now for transforming me into what You desire. Amen.

* * *

Manifest the Harvest – Try These!

__HOME CARDIO WORKOUT__
60-second Quick Feet (run in place)
20 Jump Squats (modifications are acceptable)
20 Push-ups (modifications are acceptable)
25 Bicycles
15 Mountain Climbers (modify w/ chair if needed)
REPEAT 3x's
Minimal rest in between (30-45 second)

__MJ's Favorite Recipe #7__
Quinoa Greek Salad

Ingredients for each prepared salad: ¼ cup of cooked quinoa; ½ cucumber cubed; 2 medium tomatoes; ¼ small red onion chopped; 2 tbsp of cubed feta cheese; 5 kalamata olives; ½ cup fresh spinach (or oregano leaves if you're fancy LOL!)

Ingredients for the dressing: ½ cup of olive oil; 2 lemons squeezed; ½ cup of Dijon mustard; Italian herbs (Aldi); sprinkle of salt and pepper to taste. Shake in a mason jar and use 2 tbsp per salad only.

1. Cook quinoa according to the package directions. Once done, set it aside to cool.
2. In a medium mason jar or meal prep bowl, layer your salad as follows: dressing on the bottom, cucumber, tomatoes, quinoa, onion, feta, olives, greens. Close your jar or bowl and store in the fridge until lunch time!
3. Feel free to add 4 oz of sautéed chicken per salad if you just *need* meat.

YOU'VE CHOSEN DAY SIXTEEN OF TWENTY-ONE!

DAY SIXTEEN

There's money in the masses.

I love, love, LOVE food. All kinds. Doesn't matter the type: Soul food, Greek food, Asian food, All American food, Italian food, Puerto Rican food, Mexican food (I could possibly live on tacos), food! Food is so wonderful in all its ways. Oh wait--that is the Lord, not food!

One day, I decided to do inventory of where my money was going. What a very, very bad yet great idea that was! I was outdone by the amount of money

I was spending on eating out versus the amount I was spending on purchasing actual groceries.

It literally made me sad. So sad that I went to Wendy's to grab a bite to eat and think about the fact that I was yet again sitting in the parking lot of a fast-food restaurant sad about the amount of money that I spent previously on food. It seems a bit ridiculous, right? Well, it was! But it was what I was used to doing. Not addressing the real issues of stewardship kept me on a hamster wheel with no progress.

I figured I loved food. I had the money to go and eat where I wanted when I wanted. What was the big deal? Truth is I was the BIG deal. My body was bigger than I really wanted it to be. The level of my unhappiness was too BIG to really be measured. I had really BIG cholesterol numbers. Yet, my savings account was not as BIG as I hoped.

When we think of stewardship most times, it is all about money. It can be about finances, but that isn't the full extent of what stewardship means.

How we spend our dollars matters to God. How we steward our relationships matters to the people we love. How we steward our bodies should matter to us. How we steward our time and our thought patterns matter.

The BIG problem is we often lack the desire to steward our lives in a way that pleases God. ***Matthew 6:21 says, "For where your treasure is (your money, time), there your heart will be also." (NIV)***

When I took inventory of where my "treasure" was going, I realized that I loved food more than I loved/trusted God. I realized that I was willing to spend money on temporary satisfaction (although so stinking yummy) over continual comfort/trust in God's desire for me to live in wellness (emotionally, physically, and spiritually). I realized that I was not living a supernatural lifestyle and that I allowed the things of the world to overshadow who I was called to be.

Months later, I decided that therapy was in order. I needed to be real with myself. Figuring out the why behind my emotional, and what I'd consider "social," spending led me to unhappiness. That time in therapy was super rough. I didn't immediately give up eating fast food in the parking lot before picking up my children, or drinking a bottle of wine before bed, or overspending at restaurants with friends. It took several months of uprooting my past before being able to dwindle down my *massive* spending habits.

Today, I'd like you to consider taking the challenge of looking at your bank statements. See where your money goes. A BIGGER step is to do both your bank statements and your credit card statements (the hidden truths). Wherever you spend the most money, be it food, retail therapy, or whatever your "vice" is, will tell you where your treasure lies.

After you've done this exercise, tell someone you trust (preferably a therapist). This OUT LOUD acknowledgement of the lack of stewardship will hopefully catapult you into a season of restructuring your unproductive spending habits. There are so many tools online that can assist you with creating a budget. (I wish I had a list for you, but Google is a great start). One that I like is the Dave Ramsey method, which you can also find online.

Taking this first step will help you in the future to be a good steward of not only your money, but the treasure that is your mind, body, and soul.

* * *

CAPTIVATE THE THOUGHTS OF YOUR PAST

1. Without looking at my bank/credit card statements, what do I spend the most money on outside of necessities like rent/mortgage, utilities, bills?
2. Which of these item(s) can I feasibly start to remove from my spending habits?
3. Growing up, was food or treats a reward for good behavior? Did this pattern continue into my adulthood?
4. Can I commit to 30 days of no excess spending? If not, why? If so, when can I start?

SURRENDER THEM NOW

God, I realize that the money I earn is a gift. I know that although I work hard, it is by Your grace that my needs are provided and that I lack for nothing. Help me to do the hard work of taking inventory of my time and money. I desire to live in Your will as I know that You want me to owe no man as the Bible says in Romans 13: 8. I choose to not put food on my credit cards unless for professional use. I choose to steward my life in a way that pleases You. I thank You now that my treasure, my heart, is growing to be obedient over giving in to what my flesh (body) tells me that it needs. I give You my heart, my time, my body, and relationships. Help me to choose stewardship daily. Amen.

Menia "MJ" Johnson

YOU'VE CHOSEN DAY SEVENTEEN OF TWENTY-ONE!

DAY SEVENTEEN

It's time to get to the reality of relationships.

Ever been in a relationship that you thought was just the best gift in the entire world until a moment comes where you realize you're trapped in a nightmare?

No, just me? I totally doubt it!

In this journey of wellness, the relationships we have with people, ourselves and God matters. It is not typically taught as a child to set boundaries or good expectations in relationships.

We grow up and we have a million best friends in elementary school. Some that last and most that don't. Then something happens in high school where we are trying to fit in, or wonder if people like us, see us, and notice us. Yes, this even happens for the introverts. Adulthood sneaks up on us and that is when we understand, hopefully, that it isn't the quantity of relationships we have, but the quality of the ones we hold dear.

In the mix of maturing, it is likely that our parents weren't sitting us down to discuss what healthy relationships with people, food, ourselves, or God look like. I think few are blessed with a past that would resemble that of not only a nurturing upbringing, but one where life lessons are really taught and understood. This is especially true regarding life lessons surrounding wellness.

Many of us grew up with either money, food, or free time as a reward. I especially loved when I was allowed an extra hostess cupcake after doing something I was told. I can remember my mom buying me my own gallon of milk because I just loved it so much! And if we had strawberry powder to mix in the milk, it was almost like Christmas on any given day!

Often, we use statements like, "I deserve this," and then that becomes an unhealthy habit. This is true not just for food, but in relationships too. We can then even move towards behaviors that turn people (spouses, family, close friends, etc.) away because of our co-dependency on the unproductive habits we've created. I am not saying it isn't okay to be rewarded every now and again. What I am saying is that when we've allowed ourselves to believe that over-indulgence is acceptable, this is where we find ourselves in an internal nightmare.

Relationship inventory is one of the most important parts of growing in wellness. It is imperative to understand when our habits of unproductive eating began. Who was around when it started? What events were happening in our lives at the time, and how we are currently treating those around us who appear to be against what we've allowed ourselves to need.

It isn't a wonder that there is a high level of divorce and even many who choose to walk away from the God of their youth. We have been taught and adopted the mentality that what we do matters more than what is productive, right, and sustaining.

Setting internal boundaries is one of the most important skills we can acquire as we mature in the knowledge of wellness.

Now, let us not confuse the word boundaries with completely disregarding the heart of others. They matter too. In setting internal boundaries with people, we can do this in a way that is productive and not in anger. The Bible encourages us to not sin in our anger. I've seen boundary setting gone so wrong. Let this no longer be acceptable friends.

When we consider the word sin, this is not just in how we respond to others, but how we respond to ourselves. Gluttony is sinful. When we "reward" ourselves a bit too often, or emotionally eat to the point of gluttonous behavior, we are not honoring God. We are not honoring our bodies. We are not respecting ourselves. And quite honestly, we will eventually end up in a place of being out of control in many areas of our lives due to our lack of discipline, accountability, and surrender to God.

* * *

CAPTIVATE THE THOUGHTS OF YOUR PAST

1. What is my first memory of being rewarded with food?
2. How has my lack of discipline affected my relationship with food, God, and people?
3. What relationships are currently being affected by my unproductive thought patterns and habits?
4. How can I begin to set productive internal boundaries? (with food, myself, and others)
5. Who do I need to forgive from your past or present day that has caused me to live with hidden anger?
6. How has the lack of discipline affected my relationship with God?

SURRENDER THEM NOW

Heavenly Father, thank You for seeing me and still loving me. I thank You that Your promise to me is to never leave me or forsake me according to Hebrews 13:5. Thank You that You are supporting me as I choose to live in discipline and neglect my inclinations for unproductive rewards that harm my mind, body and spirit. I surrender my past to You right now. I receive Your love, comfort, and care in this very moment as I release my mind from the thoughts of my past. These things, habits, people even, have no power over me any longer. I agree with Your will for my life. And when the days come that I forget this moment, bring me back to this declaration of renewed thinking. Let it not elongate into a new season of unproductive behaviors. In Your name I believe and receive healing. Amen.

Manifest the Harvest – Try These!

HOME CARDIO WORKOUT

30 Standing Wood Choppers
1-minute Quick Feet (running briskly in place)
30 Walkouts (check YouTube for example)
25 Mountain Climbers
25 Squat to Shoulder Press w/ weights or bands
REPEAT 3x's
Minimal rest in between (30-45 second)

MJ's Favorite Recipe #8
Sheet Pan Lemon & Garlic Butter Tilapia
(or chicken for the family)

Ingredients: 3-6 oz Tilapia filets; salt; pepper; 3 tbsp of low sodium gluten free soy sauce (Walmart), 1 lemon; 2 tbsp of unsalted butter melted (30 sec in microwave); ½ tbsp or more of cilantro (optional); ½ tsp of garlic powder; ½ tsp of chili powder or flakes; ½ tsp of cumin; ½ tsp of paprika; 1 crown of broccoli; 1 bunch of asparagus; 1 bag of cauliflower rice

1. Heat oven to 400 degrees.
2. Line a large baking pan with foil (always my go-to.) Spray/oil the pan for easy clean-up.
3. Place seasoned fish on the pan. In a small bowl combine soy sauce, lemon juice, melted butter and cilantro and drizzle over chicken. Bake for 10 minutes.
4. Flip your fish and now add seasoned green veggies and drizzle them with remaining sauce. Bake for another 10 minutes.
5. In the microwave, heat your cauliflower rice per the package directions.
6. Prep your bowls: 1 cup of cauliflower rice, 1 filet of fish, and veggies.

YOU'VE CHOSEN DAY EIGHTEEN OF TWENTY-ONE!

DAY EIGHTEEN

There are myths in your temptation.

As you are now aware, I grew up in a very charismatic church environment. I previously mentioned a song with words that suggested that God would not put more on us than we could bear. After many moments of biblical research, and living life to be honest, guess what?! It's a freaking MYTH! It isn't even true. The scripture doesn't "elude" to this at all. Here is what the scripture says: ***"No temptation has overtaken you except what is common to mankind. And God is faithful; he will not***

let you be tempted beyond what you can bear. But when you are tempted, he will also provide a way out so that you can endure it. 1 Corinthians 10:13 NIV

Shall we unpack this a bit? Yes. Yes, we should!

The first line of that scripture in the Common English Bible reads, "No temptation has seized you." What does "seized" mean? To take hold of suddenly or forcibly.

Some things can happen to us suddenly. Illness, some death occasions, car accidents, being stung by a bee, or getting an eyelash stuck in our eye while we're driving. But many things cannot. Like a broken relationship. Weight gain. Being written up at work for slacking off. In terms of wellness, it is time that causes the steady gain of weight, depression, broken relationships and so much more. God didn't put this on us. We did or circumstances around us birthed unproductive behaviors.

We must be so careful to not confuse phrases with what the Gospel means.

Let's now look at "...he won't allow you to be tempted beyond your abilities." Whoa! What are our abilities? What does this even mean? Why would He allow us to be tempted in the first got dang on place? That isn't very nice!

Welp friends, our abilities revolve around our level and measure of faith in relationship with who He is. If we allow ourselves to REALLY take inventory of the "temptations" we've experienced in our lives, what moment, if any, did we YIELD to said temptation and lean not on our own understanding (will) but align ourselves with self-control?

If there was no pause, it is likely that our ability, strength, and desire to live a harvest lifestyle, yielded to obedience is nonexistent or a bit faulty.

God has promised to ALWAYS give us a way out when we're faced with temptation. He gifted us with the Holy Spirit to live in us when we accepted Him as our Lord and Savior. The Holy Spirit lives within us to give us comfort and direction.

This gift, this promise can be used in every kind of temptation. Even in wellness. Especially when we long to be well.

I can remember the first moment I allowed my heart to yield to obedience when out to eat with friends. I had chosen for a season to give up wine.

Yes, you read that right! Wine! I love a good dark bold red wine, okay! Everyone around me ordered a glass. They offered to buy me a glass (thinking potentially that I was just being cheap), but I declined immediately. Let me tell you, I was shocked! But I felt God nudge my heart with a "thank you for being obedient." It has been a long journey of choosing to undergird my faith and live yielded to the Holy Spirit. Is it easy? No sir, no ma'am. Have I failed? Absolutely! But what I have gained over the last few years is more faith, more desire, and more ability to be yielded when temptation comes.

This has even transformed my speech and how I respond to hard situations. I could curse really well at one point in my life and tear a person's ego to shreds! I would not even care if they were hurt! They deserved it right? Uhm. Well. Let me move on.

What am I getting to here? I want to let you know that you too can live a life of harvest yielding to temptations. Will it take some practice? Yes. Will you need to build your faith muscles? Yes. Will you also need to learn new levels of discipline? Absolutely.

God *will* allow hard things to come into our lives. Some of these hard things can even feel suffocating. BUT! He promises to give us a way out of each hard circumstance that comes our way. Let us not confuse this way out to be sprinkled in fairy dust and rainbows either. Oftentimes the way out sucks and feels even harder than being in a hard situation. However, even in that, He is with us and again, has provided a gift, the Holy Spirit to bring comfort to our lives, if we choose to allow it.

* * *

CAPTIVATE THE THOUGHTS OF YOUR PAST

1. What quotes or phrases have you lived by that potentially contradict the gospel?
2. How often do you find yourself tempted by foods, adultery, pornography, laziness, or self-sabotage?

3. Do you believe in the gift that is the Holy Spirit? If no, what are your questions/concerns? Who can you confide in or receive understanding from within your circle of influence?
4. How would you measure your level of faith on a scale of 0-10? If your faith levels are low, know that it is okay, and God is still sovereign! Ask God to increase your faith and understanding of the Gospel as you digest the truth in the Bible. If you score yourself a 10, consider taking inventory of your *ability* to yield often. What areas do you need to strengthen your faith?

SURRENDER THEM NOW

Jesus, I thank you now for being with me as I complete and receive the truths of today's devotional. I appreciate that you have not given up on me and that you desire to see me live in full wellness. Help me to receive the Holy Spirit fully into my life as I desire to live a yielded lifestyle. Thank you for helping me pause before making any decisions that are unproductive to my body, mind, and spirit. I ask that you surround me with people of God centered influence to keep me accountable in the days ahead. I choose to surrender the belief that quotes and phrases that don't align with your word, are absolute truth. Thank you for replacing those words with the knowledge of the gospel that is sure to sustain me in the days ahead. Amen

YOU'VE CHOSEN DAY NINETEEN OF TWENTY-ONE!

DAY NINETEEN

Matters of the heart matter.

If you don't know me personally, you don't know that I had open heart surgery over six years ago. I was barely in my thirties when this crisis arrived in my life. It was sudden to me and those around me, but not to God or the doctors who treated me.

There was a navel orange sized tumor in my heart that broke off into my blood system and caused the circulation in my hands and feet to dwindle. My fingers turned blue and so did several of my toes. Of course, I was living day to day not knowing that something fatal was happening inside of my body. During this time, I was on the first of many "journeys" to losing some unwanted pounds, and I knew that I was not necessarily giving it my all, but I was still losing weight. *Score!* I was so happy with how quickly pounds were dropping. Little did I know that my heart rate consistently being at peak levels as if I was doing cardio, due to a tumor, was the cause.

You see, I thought it was all sudden! But it was weeks, maybe even months, of small happenings inside of my body that led to that "sudden" and necessary surgery that changed my life.

The night that I was admitted into the hospital, I laid in the hospital bed with the thought that in a few hours I would be on an operating table with my chest cracked open and a high possibility of death. Yet, through all of that, I received a revelation.

I was newly "boo'd" up with my now husband after just a few weeks of dating. My heart, not my physical heart, but my emotional heart needed healing from my past. I began to pray and God, in His grace, revealed to me that just like the time it took for the tumor to grow, the bitterness in my heart had also grown. I needed emotional surgery. I needed to acknowledge that I was broken. I had to see how I allowed parts of me to break off into people, things, foods, and unproductive habits for years!

Now, I also thought to myself, *"God, you're doing a bit much here, don't You think? I could potentially die tomorrow morning, but You want me to do all of this reflecting too?"* The nerve!

But that moment, just a few hours before surgery, changed my perspective on the matters of the heart.

Time and time again, we allow ourselves to be broken and scattered out into the lives of others. We also give into continual unproductive habits that interrupt the circulation of wellness to our minds, bodies, and spirits.

At some point in our lives, we too will face the necessity of an emotional surgery to remove the past and receive wholeness.

The Bible employs us to receive the peace of God because it will keep our hearts and minds safe (Philippians 4:7). When we surrender (allow the emotional surgery) our past behaviors, disappointments, broken relationships, unproductive habits, and lack of trust in who God is to and for us, we will awaken into the reality of grace.

For it is by grace, that we are saved, healed, rescued and whole.

No matter who hurt you or who has caused you to create habits that are unproductive to your full wellness, God wants to heal your heart. For your heart is where your decisions are truly made. Will you allow Him in today?

* * *

CAPTIVATE THE THOUGHTS OF YOUR PAST

1. Who is the first person that "broke" my heart? Am I still in relationship with them today? If so, how has that relationship changed for the better or worse?

2. What decisions (or persons) from my past have caused bitterness to build as a callus in my heart?
3. Am I at a place of being able to surrender them (people or things) and forgive? Why or why not?
4. If needed, am I able to acquire counseling to address some of the matters of my heart? When will I schedule my appointment? (Please be sure to not wait more than 24 hours.)

<u>SURRENDER THEM NOW</u>

Father, today's devotional was not easy. Help me to be willing to continue this journey of full wellness as I address the matters of my heart. I desire to love and live fully without bitter build up in the days ahead. Thank You for promising to give me peace as I trust You in this process. Amen.

* * *

Manifest the Harvest – Try These!

HOME CARDIO WORKOUT

Take a 30-minute walk or jog today (outdoors, weather permitting) or on a treadmill. Pop in your earbuds and listen to your favorite worship music.

MJ's Favorite Recipe #9
All Things Green Salad

Ingredients: 2 bags of sweet butter lettuce; 1 bag of baby spinach; 3 green apples diced; small bag of walnuts; 1 small red onion sliced; 1 small container of low-fat fetta (*optional* use only 1 tbsp per salad); low-fat vinaigrette of choice (try Aldi's raspberry vinaigrette) only use 2 tbsp of dressing per salad.

1. Prepare 3 days of salads using as much of the lettuce and spinach you'd like. You will be okay not having meat in this salad so make sure you're adding enough greens to fill you up.
2. Please drink 16 oz of water with this meal. 8 oz before and 8 oz during.

Menia "MJ" Johnson

YOU'VE CHOSEN DAY TWENTY OF TWENTY-ONE!

DAY TWENTY

Discouragement will come, but you can overcome it.

Not everyone will be in your "amen corner" rooting you on as you grow in wellness. This is the reality of growth, friend.

And it is likely that some of these people may be the ones closest to you. *Yes. This. Is. Just. Awful.*

I remember thinking to myself, *"I'm going to give updates to my family and friends all of the time! "They're going to be so proud of me!"* But the reality was some didn't even respond to text messages. Some even asked, "Why are you doing this?" Statements like: "You're doing the most." "You're going to look sick if you keep losing weight." "Weight training is going to make you look like a man."

Almost immediately, I felt discouraged. Not seen. Not loved. Not supported.

But I had to choose. Who am I desiring to please here? Them? Me? Or God? And honestly, at first, it was all about the "likes" and hand claps! I used to live off the spotlight idea. If I wasn't pleasing people, I assumed I wasn't trying hard enough or that I wasn't worth being paid attention. This too was a process of growth that took many years of therapy and restructuring of my childhood thought patterns.

When we really decide that we want to live a harvest lifestyle, we must choose to live it for God. And when we choose this, our lives are forever changed. If anyone is impacted because of the changes we make in our lives, that is a bonus and really should be a testament of God's faithfulness.

There will be many moments that discouragement will rear its ugly face. However, we can choose how it will impact our progress. Romans 5:3 reminds us that we should take pride in our problems because various kinds of trouble produces a beautiful endurance in us.

I encourage you to take these moments by the horn and then lay them at the altar! Pray about them when you're running, lifting, eating well, or meditating on scripture! This practice of continual surrender produces endurance as you grow in wellness.

Be quick to forgive those that are negative towards your goals.

Pray for their hearts to come into the knowledge of Christ in wellness.

Be slow to speak *(or curse them out)*! ***Understand this, my dear brothers and sisters: You must all be quick to listen, slow to speak, and slow to get angry." James 1:19 (NLT)***

Remember that God desires you to live in wellness, especially your spirit! ***". . . enjoy good health and that all may go well with you, even as your soul is getting along well." 3 John 1:2 (NIV)***

I have written these scriptures written out on note cards. Some are posted in my bathroom. Others on my refrigerator, and some as note cards within my journal that I carry with me.

You must be prepared spiritually and emotionally for the trials and discouragement that may come. If you aren't, you will neglect the past days of this devotional and sink back into habits and areas where you've prayed for God's assistance.

I believe in you! But most importantly, God has your back! He is with you. Loves you. He sees your progress. And has aligned the right circles of influence to come into your life either now or in the days ahead.

* * *

CAPTIVATE THE THOUGHTS OF YOUR PAST

1. Who was the first person in my life to discourage me? What happened and how did it make me feel?

2. How has this first experience impacted my life and thought patterns?
3. Who in my life today (if applicable) either discourages me or speaks against my ability to succeed (not just in wellness)? How does that make me feel?
4. What practices or boundaries can I set in place to help me not digest or internalize negative behaviors from discouragement?

SURRENDER THEM NOW

Dear God, thank You for the times of trial, for the ones who have discouraged me in the past or in my present life. Thank You that their words have no authority or power over my mind, heart, or decisions. I pray that You would silence their words of discouragement in the days to come. Thank You for my circle of influence that is current or coming in the days ahead to keep me accountable. I pray that You would allow me the strength to not give in to unproductive thoughts based on their words or even my own. Help me to remember that I am fearfully and wonderfully made. I thank You for making me in Your image and giving me a burden for what breaks Your heart. Help me to be quick to forgive and slow to anger in the days ahead. I praise You for Your sovereignty in my life. I honor You today, tomorrow, and in the days to come with my body, my mind, and my spirit. Amen.

YOU'VE CHOSEN DAY TWENTY-ONE OF TWENTY-ONE!

DAY TWENTY-ONE

What now?

You have successfully completed TWENTY-ONE DAYS of self-evaluation through a guided, biblical devotional! I am so proud of you! Way to be consistent!

Now, what will you do tomorrow?

Here are a few options:

*If you're feeling like you weren't fully dialed into this process. Start over! Starting over is totally a thing and there is no shame in acknowledging that you may not have been fully engaged for twenty-one days.

When you start over (if applicable), please be sure to take no more than 7 days to begin again. You want to be sure that you're all in this next go around! Get yourself a new journal because you just never know the new revelations you'll discover since you're a bit more open to the process.

*Create a daily schedule for yourself! Planning your day will decrease the amount of unproductive food choices and/or missing an opportunity to move your body, and have moments of prayer time

When creating your schedule, be sure you're also including two days to plan what your meals will be. If you're a person who travels often, be sure to scope out the land of healthy eating options where you'll be! This only takes a few minutes! (Don't be lazy! You can do this!)

*Get yourself an accountability partner or join a wellness group that aligns with your goals

*Pray! There is so much power in the habit of daily prayer. Not just to ask God to be your magical genie and do things for you, but to thank Him, praise

Him and spend some time simply acknowledging His power and authority in and around your life.

*Set timers on your phone to help you remember to get in your water! When I first started this whole "get in your water" situation, I set an alarm on my cell for the half hour mark of every hour of my workday (9-5) to drink 12-16 oz of water. I add lemon or fresh fruit often to get it in!

*Reconcile Relationships: You should only venture into an in-person conversation if you feel the peace and nudge of God. Not every moment of reconciliation requires an in-person meeting. Be yielded!

*Schedule weekly, monthly, or quarterly therapy sessions to help you maintain your decision to live in wellness. Remember, seeing a therapist doesn't mean that your life is falling apart! It simply means that you're attentive to your mental health. ***Proverbs 15:22*** states, ***"Plans fail for lack of counsel, but with many advisers they succeed." (NIV)***

*Set a visit with a nutritionist and allergist before you decide to go with any "fad" diets. Not every person is meant to be vegan, vegetarian or go on a low carb diet. It is important that you know what your body needs, can tolerate, and responds to.

*If you don't already have a body of faith believers (church, small group) please consider finding a place where your heart and spirit can be fed with the Gospel of Christ. Again, not every building that says it is a church is teaching the gospel. So, this too is a matter of prayer. God is so dope that He cares about this too! ***"For where two or three gather in my name, there am I with them." Matthew 18:20 NIV***

GO BANANAS! Begin with setting ATTAINABLE bi-monthly goals. Write them down! And stay the course! Remember: God is the one who directs your path as you plan to crush your goals. ***"A man's heart plans his way, but the Lord directs his steps. Proverbs 16:9 NKJV***

After you write out those goals, better yet, before you write them out, pray about them. Then write them down. Ask God to honor your desire **and** consistent execution to be disciplined and yielded.

*Lastly, do not fear. If you've set out to start something new in the past and failed mid-way, that can end today. The fear of success is a real thing! And in that, there potentially is a rooted issue from your past that needs some attention. ***"For God has not given us a spirit of fear and timidity, but of power, love, and self-discipline." 2 Timothy 1:7 NLT*** (Write this on a note card and place it on your nightstand or bathroom mirror.

* * *

CAPTIVATE THE THOUGHTS OF YOUR PAST

1. What fears do I have of succeeding? (not just in wellness)
2. By what date will I set my daily schedule? (Please do not let this go longer than 24-48 hours after the completion of this devotional.)
3. What is the name of the person I trust the most to hold me accountable in the days ahead? When will I ask their permission/availability to keep me accountable?

SURRENDER THEM NOW

Jesus! Thank you! Thank you for being my provider. My counselor. My friend. My way maker. My healer. My Savior. It is only because of You that my mind is and has been renewed. Thank You for caring about my wellness. I thank You for creating my parents who created me. Thank You for the functioning of my limbs, my mind, and growing my soul into a yielded space that the Holy Spirit dwells. Thank You for promising to never leave me or forsake me. I praise You because You simply are, the Great I am! The Prince of Peace! The Mighty Most High God. It is only by Your grace that I am saved. Thank You for directing my path, my goals, and even digesting every productive meal in the days ahead. I honor Your name in living a harvest lifestyle. Amen.

* * *

Manifest the Harvest – Try These!

<u>HOME CARDIO WORKOUT</u>
60 Second Skaters
30-seconds of Jumping Rope
(You don't need a rope to do this!)
25 Squats
20 Push-ups
20 Russian Twists
REPEAT 3x's

<u>MJ's Favorite Recipe #9</u>
Courageous Curry Chickpea Bowl

Ingredients:1 pound of lean ground turkey; 1 bag of cauliflower rice; 2 crowns of broccoli; 3 tbsp. of curry powder; 3 teaspoons of minced garlic in oil; 1 tbsp. of pink salt; ½ lemon

1. Brown ground turkey.
2. In a large saucepan, add your minced garlic in oil and simmer for 30 seconds.

3. In a large pan, pour ½ cup of water in and add your broccoli. Steam for 8 minutes, then top with a squeeze of lemon and the remainder of your pink salt.
4. Heat your frozen cauliflower in a pan, add remainder of the curry powder, and a sprinkle of salt and pepper to taste.
5. Now portion your chickpeas out to 4 oz (or ½ cup if using a measuring cup).
6. Prep your bowl: 1 cup of cauliflower, 1 cup of broccoli and 1 cup of ground turkey

RESOURCES

Things from the earth that encourage good health and weight maintenance:

TURMERIC
According to studies, turmeric can help your body burn fat. In the study, there were two groups of mice, one was fed curcumin while the other wasn't. The results were that the group of mice that had curcumin lost more weight than the other group that did not have it. Turmeric (which was derived from curcumin and is essentially the same thing) is a warming spice; it increases the body heat which can boost your metabolism and provide other health benefits.

CINNAMON

Cinnamon is said to curb hunger cravings, control blood sugar level and make you feel fuller for longer. You can add cinnamon to your oatmeal, mix it in yoghurt or put it in your tea. It is also a great addition to meat and chicken.

CAYENNE PEPPER

Cayenne pepper raises the body temperature which boosts your metabolism. The higher the metabolism, the more calorie you burn. Adding this spice to your meal can help you burn up to 100 calories per meal. You can sprinkle cayenne pepper on nuts, soup, eggs, and dips for that extra kick.

ROSEMARY

Rosemary helps to increase your metabolic rate. It also aids digestion and weight loss. These green pointed leaves are to be soaked in boiling water for a few minutes. The strained water can be consumed lukewarm at any time of the day but not empty stomach.

CARDAMOM

Cardamom, also called elaichi, is a popular Indian spice with a unique flavor. It is thermogenic in nature and that is why it helps you in losing weight. It also prevents the formation of gas, which makes you feel bloated and uneasy. You can add a pinch or two of cardamom powder to your food to lose weight faster.

BLACK PEPPER

How can we not mention black pepper while talking about Indian spices! Cousin to cayenne pepper, black pepper is rich in piperine, which gives black pepper its unique flavor. This one ingredient prevents the formation of fat cells and thus, helps you to lose, and later maintain, that weight. One can combine black pepper and cayenne pepper for better weight loss results!

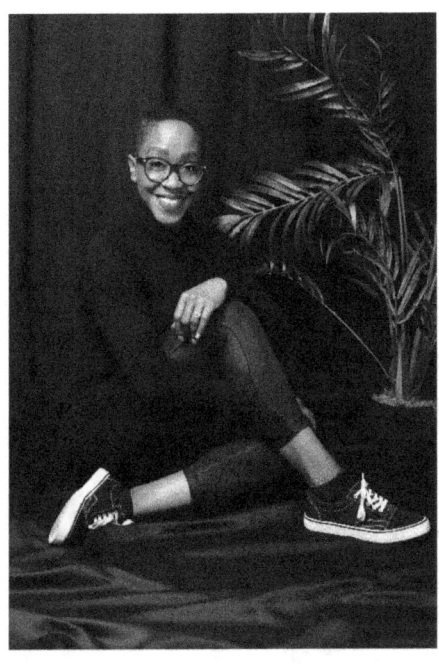

Menia "MJ" Johnson is a faith-based accountability and wellness coach who helps men and women uproot the patterns of their past to live in wellness: mind, body, and spirit.

Before writing about wellness, she began her own journey that combined therapy, nutrition, and physical fitness. Since then, MJ has helped hundreds of people discover wellness through meal planning, fitness classes, and online accountability coaching to elevate minds, spirits, and bodies to a new level of discipline. Most recently, MJ placed third in a body building bikini competition as a personal goal and tool to spread the Gospel of Jesus to athletes in the industry.

While she thoroughly enjoys wellness being a part of her life, MJ also holds the position of Assistant Vice President of Lending at Renovo Financial providing capital for real estate developers in Chicago IL. She is also a wife, mother of 4, and a grandmother of one beautiful baby girl. She also holds the position of Co-Founder of Anthem Fit Life Group of Anthem Church in Hammond, Indiana.

God has always been the center of her life, and many would characterize her as a "Christian Hippie" because she is a very free-spirited and energetic!

Menia "MJ" Johnson can be found on Instagram at ***@mjfaith2fitness*** for daily inspiration and privately messaged there for accountability opportunities.

www.ingramcontent.com/pod-product-compliance
Lightning Source LLC
Chambersburg PA
CBHW070908080526
44589CB00013B/1222